Belly Fat Diet
Secrets to Losing Fat without Eating Less: Natural and Effective Ways to Lose Belly Fat

Simon Roche

Finicky, Inc.

New York

Lose Belly Fat: Healthy and Effective Ways to Burn Fat Even If You're Busy

About me

FREE Bonus: [https://healthresultswealth.wordpress.com/ **]**
Motivational Coffee

Hi, my name is Simon Roche, Founder of "Finicky.us" and also the author to many entrepreneurial and self-help books.

I have seen that I was different since I was a kid. When other kids wanted to play, I wanted to be productive and better myself. Not to say that I didn't play on my free time, I just didn't play longer than I needed. I always set my expectations out of my reach and I truly hope that my readers do the same. I have visited many companies during my career and I can say that I have learned more than if I were to have worked for a company.

As a thank you for considering my book, I will provide you with one of my many experiences while visiting a friend at Google. My friend who was previously the "Strategic Partner Lead" at Google has had many accomplish through his career and no longer works at Google. We became friends in our marketing course and have still kept in contact.

He gave me a tip about the process of hiring people for my company. During the selection process, he weaves out many strong candidates. Why? Simply because they aren't smarter than me, the interviewer. He explains that if you want a good company, then you surround yourself with average brains that just want to get by. At Google, we don't want average, we want the smartest. Smart people hire smarter people and that's how Google is still on top of its industry. He stated, "I want to hire someone who is smarter than me, works better than me, and is more innovative than me. That way I will be happy when they take my position, as I move on to another chapter in my life"

Through my books, I will share many of my unique experiences and will provide you with mistakes that I have made myself as an entrepreneur.

information is without contract or any type of guarantee assurance.

The trademarks that are used are without any consent, and the publication of the trademark is without permission or backing by the trademark owner. All trademarks and brands within this book are for clarifying purposes only and are the owned by the owners themselves, not affiliated with this document.

Words from the Author

Before you start reading this book, I will need you to keep a thought in mind.

"To be able to sacrifice what you are, for who you will become"

In other words, if you put aside your excuses, you will get the results you have always wanted. It's time to make a decision. You can choose to stay the way you are or you can decide to take steps towards change.

No one is stopping you from where you want to go, the only person that is stopping you is YOU. Remind yourself every day of who you want to be, and remember to make the right decisions towards your goal. One way to keep your goals set is by checking up on yourself at the end of each week. Set a goal for 2 pounds each week, and by the end of the month you will have cut 8 pounds. Keep your short-term goals small so that it is achievable, but keep your long-term goals big, so that there is no ceiling towards your success.

Belly Fat: How to Lose Belly Fat in 10 Days

Introduction

Before reading on, keep in mind that this book will be able to guide you to your goal of losing belly fat and living a healthy life. The routines provided will become natural and you're brain and body will feel awake by the end of these 10 days. This book will be your health coach, but it is up to you to decide if you want to see change. I can show you the way

Do we do it out of vanity or are we really concerned about our health? This is the number one question when it comes to wanting to lose the ever stubborn belly fat. In America alone, there are over 300 diets that promise to give you rock-hard abs, but this begs the question – How come America is still one of the fattest countries?

To answer the first question, getting in shape will boost your confidence and give you a positive physical change. So whether you;

- Want to rock a summer bikini
- Are tired of being a lazy bum
- Want to make a positive change
- Want to secure your health
- Want to fit in your favorite skinny jeans
- Have a wedding coming up
- Want to regain your youthful good looks
- Were ready to make a change like yesterday but need the motivation...the list is endless.

Whatever your scenario, we have the solution!

Let's face it, losing belly fat is no walk in the park, it is really, really hard and with summer time around the corner, the pressure to fit into our swim suits is on. Most of us relish the thought of sun bathing on white sandy beaches, sipping on our favorite cocktails. But sadly, the bulge gets in the way of this dream. Now, it is important to note that belly fat is not merely a wardrobe malfunction it's much deeper than 'vanity'. Yes, we all want to display washboard abs in your monokini and bikinis but, belly fat is a **MAJOR** health problem.

We all have fat around our major organs that provide cushioning against shocks. The problem comes in when this fat (visceral fat)is too much as it can now interfere with how our organs function and result in serious health conditions such as heart disease, diabetes, cancers, stroke and so on. This is one of the reasons why you need to work on your tummy.

We also want to help kick start your journey to your ideal body with this 10 day program that will leave you feeling better than ever before. Whether you are doing it for 'vanity' or health reasons, what I can guarantee you are immense confidence and happiness once you complete this 10 day program, which of course doesn't end there!

As for the second question, most of us can attest to following at least one diet plan that may or may have not given us the results we were looking for. You may have had of the 80/20 rule:

80 Percent Dieting + 20% Physical Exercise = 100% Healthy Body

Or the 120 rule:

You can eat anything you want for as long as you exert your body at 120%

I am not going to utterly dismiss any of these rules, but from my own experience and those of close friends, I have come to find that 100% commitment to a healthy lifestyle is your safest bet for your dream body in the shortest time possible.

What does 100% commitment to a healthy lifestyle entail?

- The food you eat
- The strength training you do
- The high intensity interval training you do
- The low impact interval training you do
- The amount of rest and sleep you get
- The amount of work/ study you get done
- Your social life – how you interact with others
- The time you spend meditating or connecting to a higher power.

All these aspects will make or break your weight loss efforts and we are going to show you exactly how to get started on these so you can lose belly fat quickly and also maintain your new hot body!

One Size Does Not Fit All!

In a world where you see your favorite icon, who is in her mid-forties, rocking a toned and lean body, better than what you had as a teenager; there is certainly a lot of pressure to lose belly fat and look the part. What most of us don't understand or refuse to admit, is that there is no single 'one size fits all, belly fat loss approach' that works in the same way for all of us. Let us look at the following scenario to demystify this approach.

It's been about 6 years since you linked up with your campus bff who you had been struggling together with weight issues ever since you became buddies. She one day calls to inform you she has a job interview in your state and she will pass by for a visit. You are obviously over the moon because it's been an eternity since you last saw each other. Come D-day, you go pick her up at the airport and a stunning lady who doesn't look a day past 20 comes beaming at you and gives you a very warm hug and even calls you by your pet name...

To cut the long story short, your bff tells you of a great new diet that she has been following and how she managed to lose 10 pounds in only 2 weeks and she further tells you it only took her six months to move from a size 18 to a size 4. You can't believe your eyes because all along you knew diets were fads aimed at robbing you of your money and self-esteem but then standing before you is living proof that dieting actually works.

With the new found motivation, you clean up your pantry and stock up on the recommended foods by your new diet and you have already snapped a mental picture of how you are going to look in 2 weeks, 3 months all up to 6 months. However, 3 days on to the diet and you start experiencing intense stomach pains and you hit up your friend to ask if it's normal. She tells you she didn't experience that but assures you that people are different - this should have been your cue to stop immediately. But, you push on because you already have a picture of yourself 6 months down the line...

Six months down the line, all you have managed to lose is 5 pounds and truck loads of self-esteem. The moral of the story is that we are all made very unique. There are so many things that have been said about the best weight loss strategies some of which are true while others are utter gibberish. In this book, we are hoping to shed some light on this matter so you can focus on **YOUR** own **GOALS**.

To start with, you should not be seduced by the allure of wanting to look like so and so. Your goal should be specifically tailored to your needs and not a certain idealistic figure, individual or image. Your end goal should be geared towards happiness that you are going to experience by being healthy. This doesn't mean that you have to be a size zero to be happy.

We have different body types, different genes, different body chemistry and different goals. In this book, our aim is to bring together all these variations into very realistic and achievable end goals within the shortest time possible – one month!

1. How to make the program fit any fitness level you are at

But I am overweight, unfit and have never exercised before...

OKAY – there is no better time to start than now!

Embracing a healthy lifestyle is essential for everyone – whether you are a gym bunny, cross fit trainer or even if you have never trained a day in your life. Losing weight feels like someone has literally lifted a huge mountain off your back. It allows you to experience clarity of mind, fills you with vitality and happiness like you never knew before and that is why we are focused on kick starting your weight loss journey by introducing you to healthy living standards.

For this 10 day period where we embark to kick start your healthy living, we are going to focus on three main styles of training:

Resistance/ strength/ weight training

In a nutshell, resistance training is based on the science that says your muscles will work to prevail over a resistant force when required to do so. When you do this on a regular basis, your muscles become stronger. Other benefits of resistance training are; improved bone density, joint function, and ligament and tendon strength.

Cardiovascular (cardio) training

Basically, cardio training is any form of exercise that quickly raises your heart beat. These exercises are based on the fact that our bodies are typically made to move and so to keep your muscles in shape, you need to move them.

Cardio training makes your heart stronger and also improves the delivery of oxygen to your lungs and all the cells in your body.

Stretching/ warm up

This involves training that stretches muscle fibers so as to increase the flexibility of your muscles and tendons, improve motion, and prevent injuries especially during resistance and cardio training.

These three training styles are your keys to fast and sustainable weight loss and after this one month, you are going to record massive improvement.

2. Why adding weights makes a difference

Training using weights is the fastest way to lose belly fat. Weight training targets fast twitch muscle fibers that use up a lot of calories. If you use up more calories than you are eating, you are definitely going to see results and **YES**, using weights makes all the difference.

3. What kind of results you should see

Weight loss

It won't be long before clothes start feeling a bit loose and this is a sure sign that you are doing something right. Keep up with the training and you are sure to see more and more results.

Improved mood

When you engage in physical activity, this triggers the release of some feel good chemicals from your brain such as dopamine and serotonin that leave you feeling more relaxed and happier. By the end of this 10 day program, you should have a very positive image about yourself which will in turn improve your self-esteem and also your confidence.

Increased energy

Feeling winded after performing your normal daily activities or going up a flight of stairs? Then you are definitely in the right place! A combination of strength training, cardio and stretching is the best antidote for fatigue and loss of energy. These exercises take oxygen and essential nutrients right into your tissues and also help your cardiovascular system to work in a more efficient way. With a heart and a pair of lungs that work efficiently, you will have unending pockets of energy.

Sleeping beauty

Do you toss and turn for hours unending before finally falling asleep only for your alarm to ring 3 hours later? With the three training techniques, this is going to be past tense. A word of caution is not to train right before bedtime as you will be too pumped up to sleep.

Steamy sex life

If before you felt too out of shape or too tired to enjoy some intimacy with your partner, you will experience a whole 360 change. Training enhances female arousal and also helps prevent and reduces instances of erectile dysfunction in men. Additionally, it gives you the stamina to go on and on and on.

The bottom line is with this 10 day program, you are going to feel better about every aspect of your life. One piece of advice:

Take the approach of the hare when it comes to training and not that of the tortoise!

Fat – The Good, the Bad and the Ugly!

Is there such a thing as good fats? Most of us find ourselves asking ourselves this question due to the fact that all dietary fat has been demonized for the longest of time. Until recently, we were advised to eat high carb, low fat foods. The question is, if fats and oils are so bad, why are avocados good for us yet they are high in fat?

The truth is, fats are not created equally and the type of fats you consume is more important to your health than the total amount of fat in your plate, not to say that this too is not important. Instead of completely cutting out fats from your everyday life, you need to learn to make healthier choices and clever substitutions to get maximum benefit out of the good fats.

Let us now delve deeper into this concept and understand the fats we should be eating and those that we should avoid to help torch away the belly fat.

The good...

Did you know that some fats can help you get rid of your belly fat once and for all?

YES! In fact a good number of fats come with a raft of amazing health benefits such as weight loss, lowering bad cholesterol level, promoting heart health, prevention of diabetes and metabolic syndrome that is correlated to belly fat and not forgetting boosting brain health. We are talking about unsaturated fats.

Monounsaturated fats: these are plant based oils that increase your levels of good cholesterol in addition to lowering your levels of bad cholesterol, risk of stroke and heart diseases. Great sources are; canola oil, peanut oil, sunflower oil, olive oil, sesame oil, olives, avocado, peanut butter and generally all nuts.

Polyunsaturated oils: these are basically omega-3 and omega-6 essential fatty acids. Our bodies do not produce these essential oils yet they play very important roles and so we need to get them from food. These fatty acids will not only help you lower your cholesterol levels, they have also been shown to help in weight loss and particularly the weight round your waistline that never seems to budge.

Great sources are; fatty fish – tuna, salmon, mackerel, trout, herring and sardines, soybean oil walnuts, tofu, soymilk, corn oil, safflower oil, sunflower oil, pumpkin and sesame seeds.

The bad...

You should not avoid saturated fats; limit your intake to about 10% of your total dietary intake. Saturated fats have been linked to increased cholesterol levels and heart disease. These fats are found in fatty cuts of meats such as lamb, beef and pork, full-fat dairy products, dark meat in chicken and also the skin, palm oil, ice cream, lard, cheese and butter.

It is important to note that although these foods have saturated fats, they nourish your body with essential nutrients and minerals and thus should not be eliminated from your diet completely. Coconut oil has short chain saturated fats that are actually good for your health. The important thing is to make good food choices. For example opt for pastured meats, wild caught fish, organic foods and free range poultry.

The evil...

Trans fats are made using hydrogen to keep them in solid state at room temperature and are thus known as hydrogenated oils.

Trans fats can be very devastating to your body and play a very big role in causing heart related illnesses and are found in most fried and processed foods. Steer clear of foods that have the words hydrogenated, shortening or partially hydrogenated. A sure way of knowing if a food product is trans fat free is if it has less than half a gram of trans fats in every serving.

You will find trans fats in; fried food (chicken nuggets, French fries, fried chicken, breaded fish...), pizza dough, doughnuts, cookies, commercially baked pastry, packaged snack foods (chips, microwave popcorn, crackers, corn puffs...), vegetable shortening, margarine, candy bars...

The bottom line...

Some fats are a very good thing and will provide you with immense health benefits. The trick is to eat the good fats – unsaturated fats, and most importantly don't go in a rampage and eat excessive amounts.

Additionally, swap the unhealthy fats with the healthy ones when cooking and also avoid processed foods that are most liked doused in truckloads of trans fats.

True Happiness Is the Key to Melting Belly Fat

We are going to start with very important question; **what does true happiness mean to you**? But, how do you measure something as personal and intangible as happiness?

We may never get the words to define this but one thing is for sure, true happiness will forever be unmistakable. When you are happy, it becomes pretty obvious to everyone around you. You will move through life with a bright sparkle in your eyes and a spring in your step. Your contentment and positive energy will be contagious to everyone you meet.

So, let's get back to the question; **what does true happiness mean to you**?

Contrary to what we have been made to believe happiness is not about the type of car you are driving or the house you live in, the clothes you put on or any other external markers. True happiness can only come from within.

So, how will happiness help me lose this bulge?

Well, let's read on o find out.

Move that body!

Engaging your body in vigorous physical activity not only helps you torch away all the belly fat but it also helps dispel any feeling of negativity and depression. When you exercise, your brain triggers the release of hormones and neurotransmitters such as serotonin and dopamine which are feel good hormones that generate happy feelings

With exercise, you will be experiencing an all-time high 24/7 and will not need a whole tub of ice cream or a full box of cookies or chocolate to help you feel good. Additionally, people who engage in physical fitness tend to make very healthy food choices as they don't want to sabotage all the hard work they have been doing in the gym.

Exercise also improves your metabolism and immunity thus protecting you from disease. With a healthy lifestyle and a trim waist line what's to stop you from being happy? Whether you like running, dancing, rock climbing, Pilates, spinning, rowing or lifting weights; go for whatever rocks your boat!

Make smart food choices

Being overweight, having a beer gut or not eating healthy, nutritious foods can negatively impact your mood. This is most likely going to lead to a love-hate kind of relationship with your food. For example after gobbling an entire bag of chips, a whole pizza or any other 'guilty pleasure', most of us are filled with feelings of guilt and shame for not having enough will power to resist the temptation of eating the whole bag of chips. This if unchecked can turn into a vicious cycle of overeating and self-loathing which will only fuel your belly gut and flush your self-esteem down the drain.

On the contrary, if you make healthy food choices and practice mindful eating, you will be so proud of yourself for making the right food choices and even when you indulge in an occasional snack, you will be ready to stop after 2 cookies and not go all the way until you reach the bottom of your cookie jar.

In the end, your self-confidence will be so strong and your belly fat will be gone and you will now fit into your favorite jeans, you will be more than ready to go frolicking in the sand come summer with no apologies to make about your body!

Beauty sleep

We all know that getting enough sleep is paramount to staying healthy. But, your job is hanging by a single thread, your car is almost getting repossessed, you are behind on your mortgage payments, your teenage daughter is driving you nuts...how are you supposed to get any sleep?

I will start by telling you why you need to sleep for a minimum of 7 hours every single day. When you sleep, all the cells in your body recover from all the strenuous day's activities and also make necessary repairs for any damaged cells.

When you don't log in enough sleep, your brain triggers the release of adrenalin a hormone that is tasked with providing you with instant energy. This keeps you alert as you perform all
of your duties during the day. Adrenalin has to be reinforced by another hormone called cortisol, which is tasked with replenishing the used up energy so you don't feel too tired to continue with the rest of your day.

Now, the problem is this; the lives we are currently leading are pretty much sedentary and we do not use up all the energy being released by adrenalin with the help of cortisol. These two by the way, spike your hunger because we need something to provide the energy. So, you have eaten, eaten and eaten but all the energy produced cannot be used up; where does it go? Your fat pockets in your tummy, thigh, upper arms and love handles!

Incorporate exercise and healthy eating into your lifestyle and despite the many curve balls that are thrown in your way by life, you are going to do the best you can to tackle them during the day and at night, you are going to sleep like a little baby!

When you embrace happiness, you will be able to face stressful situations head on rather than succumbing to them. If life hands you lemons, you will go ahead and make the best damn lemonade you can ever get. By doing this, you will never seek to find solace in food and your wash board abs are going to thank you for it!

Pump Up Your Metabolism And Shred All The Belly Fat!

Fact: calories can never be the same! Some make you store muscle while others make you store fat!

How is this important?

Well, metabolism is the process your body utilizes energy (calories) for the various bodily functions such as repairing damaged cells to running a marathon. As such, the quality of calories will make a difference especially when all the calories have not been used up and some have to be stored. Calories from fats will be stored as fats and those from protein are going to be stored in muscle and as you know; if you exercise, your muscles burn calories even when you are just sitting down!

Exercise is one of the surest ways to boost your metabolism. Additionally, you can make wise food choices to help blast that belly fat. Here are five of the best metabolism boosting foods.

Tuna

This is an omega-3 fatty acids power house. These essential fatty acids stimulate the production of the hormone leptin that gives you the feeling of fullness thereby curbing your appetite and it also boosts your metabolism.

Ensure you get wild caught fish that has got very low incidences of mercury contamination and that has also been exposed to the natural feeing system that varies with the different seasons unlike farmed fish that are mostly fed on grains all year round. You can also substitute tuna with other wild caught fatty fish such as herring, salmon, sardines and mackerel.

Green tea

Green tea coupled with a fitness regimen makes the perfect belly fat loss recipe. This is not to say that you should not be eating any other food. Green tea contains a special chemical, epigallocatechin that stimulates your nervous system without interfering with your heart rate. What this does is increase your metabolism helping you burn a whole lot of extra calories.

About three cups of this amazing beverage will do the job just don't add any artificial additives including sugar. You an instead add a few drops of natural honey.

Rolled oats

Rolled oats make the perfect breakfast meal as they help you stave off hunger. To add to this, whole grains take more energy to digest and so you burn off calories even when eating them. You don't have to worry about running to the office vending machine to grab a snickers bar to help with the hunger midmorning; rolled oats will easily sustain you until lunch time.

Spicy hot peppers

Cayennes, habaneros, jalapenos don't just give our food a great kick, they also spice up your metabolism using capsaicin, a chemical that increases your metabolism by up to 25% for up to 3 hours after consumption. Isn't this amazing?

So don't be shy to add a little hotness into your meals, your tummy will thank you for it!

Grape fruit

This is the holy grail of citrus fruits and rightly so. It contains a powerful antioxidant, naringerin which helps your body metabolize insulin more efficiently. By keeping your blood sugar levels in check, it helps boost your metabolism by improving calorie burn which goes a long way in fighting that stubborn belly fat.

You can use grapefruit to add a bit of punch to your green salad or it as is as part of your breakfast.

Make these five foods a regular part of your meals and you are going to see a great improvement the next time you take your measurements. In addition, add foods that have a variety of color such as greens, orange and red into your meals as they are filled with antioxidants that rev up your metabolism.

The rule of thumb is to only eat natural foods; those that grow as plants and not those which are manufactured in a plant!

Tricks to Lose Belly Fat in 10 Day

Contrary to popular belief, doing a whole bunch of sit-ups and other crunches will not give you the tummy of your dreams especially if you don't make any changes in your diet. Just by changing your diet and exercise regimen will give you significant results in just 10 days! However, keep in mind that fat loss is a gradual process and these 10 days are going to give you a head start towards achieving your dream body

Cut out all the junk

Anything in your kitchen like candy, cookies, chips, crackers, cakes, doughnuts or any other thing that is high in sugar, calories cholesterol and fat should go straight to your garbage bag. Remember, if you feed your body with junk, you are going to look like junk but, if you nourish yourself with natural and healthy food, you are going to be the true picture of health.

Junk food is so aptly named because they add very little nutritional value to your meals and merely fill you up with loads of calories. With such an unhealthy diet, you are going to just maintain your weight, with your belly fat not budging.

Hydrate, hydrate and hydrate more

Staying hydrated helps your body flush out accumulated toxins in your body. Now, it is important to note that toxins usually attach themselves to fat cell, by flushing out the toxins, your body is going to be able to metabolize the fat and use it to fuel your body's activities.

Additionally, taking a glass of water before every meal will help you eat less at every meal in addition to helping ease your digestion. You will be surprised at how much reducing belly bloat will take inches off your waistline. Go for eight to ten glasses of water every day. If however you don't like the taste of plain water, you can add some punch to your water by adding lemon slices to your glass of water or fresh berries or even grapes.

Exercise for 30-45 minutes every day

Aerobic exercises will get your heart rate up and also torch away your belly fat. Swimming, dancing, biking and running are great aerobic exercise. Exercise consistently and you will take full delight in the results.

You can also incorporate strength training or weight lifting exercises which burn more calories compared to aerobic exercises. For best results, do aerobic exercises and weight lifting exercises on alternating days.

When doing weight lifting exercises, focus on those that target your abdominal and oblique muscles for a well-toned mid-section.

High fiber is always best

Veggies, whole grains, legumes, nuts and high fiber fruits are your best bet when it comes to losing belly fat. The high fiber keeps your heart healthy and also keeps you full longer helping you lose weight without being hungry and miserable. High fiber foods also help improve your bowel movements so you no longer have to worry about constipation.

Stay limber

Exercises such as yoga and Pilates work on strengthening your whole body. By working on your body's entire fitness you will increase your metabolism speed and also build muscle definition so you burn calories even when stationary. The faster you burn calories, the faster your tummy will shrink

A perfect day of eating

Combine fiber (fruits, veggies and whole grains) and protein (fish, eggs, meat, dairy and nuts) at every meal. When you eat these foods together, they take longer to digest compared to simple carbs and thus keep you full longer.

Have a small snack in between two major meals; hat is, breakfast, mid-morning, lunch, mid-afternoon and dinner. This will fuel your metabolism and help prevent binge eating and blood sugar high and lows.

Get up, drink lots of water, eat healthy and move around. Your calorie intake should fall in the range of 1550-2100; if you are super active; go towards the higher range, if not go to the lower range.

It is important to switch up your meals otherwise your metabolism is going to get used to them and slow down.

Conclusion

Let me have my last cookie, my last scoop of ice cream, my last slice of pizza, my last late of French fries...come Monday am going to fully embrace a fully healthy lifestyle... So many of us can relate to such sentiments but the question you should be asking yourself is; what if Monday never comes... what if tomorrow never comes?

The best time to start losing your belly fat is now! If you are unhappy with how your tummy looks you need to start acting right now! By this time next week, your waist will measure a few inches less and this trend will continue until you achieve you dream body.

This belly fat loss guide will help you place healthy food in the heart of your home and it will also help you enjoy the healthy lifestyle as this time you know that every bit you lake is going to have a very positive impact on your body and every time you exercise, you move closer and closer to wash board abs.

Your health is your number one priority and remember, belly fat is the worst of them all so get moving and eat healthy and all the best as you set out on this amazing journey towards achieving your dream body!

I want you to thank yourself for wanting to change and I hope you walk away inspired or smarter.

As you read on you will find tips used by entrepreneurs, and motivational thoughts that come from coaches and entrepreneurs themselves. Have Fun and good luck with your endeavors. Before moving on, I just want to remind you that we are all born on this earth as equals. Some may have more support than others, but we can only characterize ourselves by our own actions. In other words, everyone in this world has potential hidden in a box. Some choose to find a way to open it, and some just leave it there.

Think about this and try to figure out who you are.

Some may be okay living an average life, but then there are also others who constantly look for better.

Life Hacking Tips Used by the Entrepreneurs!
Coffee Nap

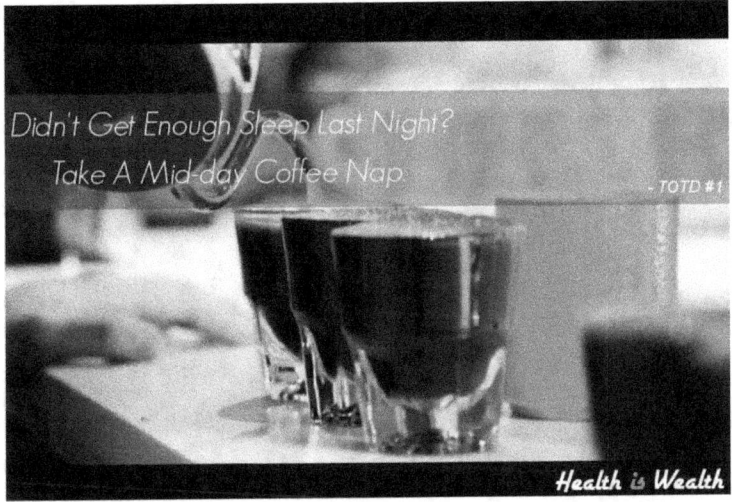

This method provided is called, "Caffeine Nap", where you drink a cup of coffee and nap for 15 minutes. The 15 minutes gives you time to rest and allows the caffeine to travel through your gastro-intestinal tract. This will provide you with a refreshing reboot by the time you wake up. But don't go over the 15-20 minutes limit or else you'll wake up in a sleepy state.

Plan the Night Before

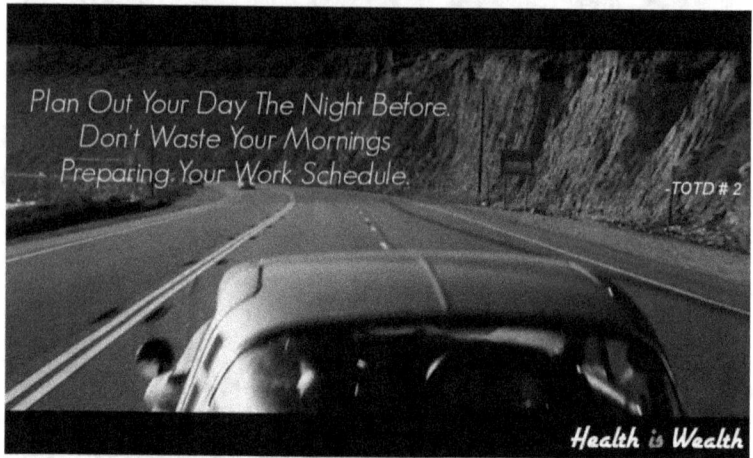

You heard of this before, you can either work hard or work smart. It's your choice. There's nothing wrong about working hard, but what's the point of working hard if the results are not there. You need to work smart and change up your routine so that your work is actually effective. Tonight before you go to bed, plan out your work for the next day so that you don't waste time in the morning. Don't waste your mornings on planning out what you want to work on as you are wasting your brains fuel. Your brain is packed with fuel from last night's rest, so go use it on something productive. Don't be like the majority of people who sit on their desk wondering what they need to do. Hope this helps!

Acknowledge Your Accomplishments, But....

You have one win in your hand, but that's not enough. It's not time to celebrate just yet. This is only a small win towards your goal. If you celebrate now, you might just lose the fire that you've always had in you to pursue your dreams. So when you reach a goal, recognize it. Please do so as it will be your source of motivation. The motivation that tells you, maybe it is possible. Maybe this dream isn't out of my reach. Just remember to set your goals high and when you do reach them, set them even higher the next time.

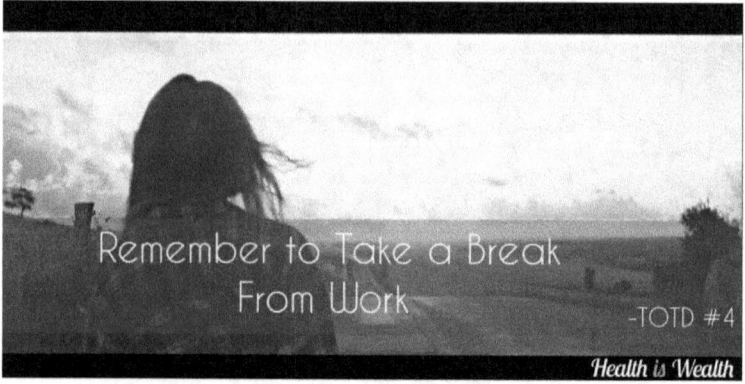

Most of us work for a living, and sometimes we work so hard that we feel too tired to spend time with the people we love. Just remember that our work will always change, but our family will always be there. On another thought, we need to take breaks during excessive periods of work, so that we can replenish our thoughts. Take a walk and get some fresh air.

Motivation for Those Who Want to Succeed
Are You Committed?

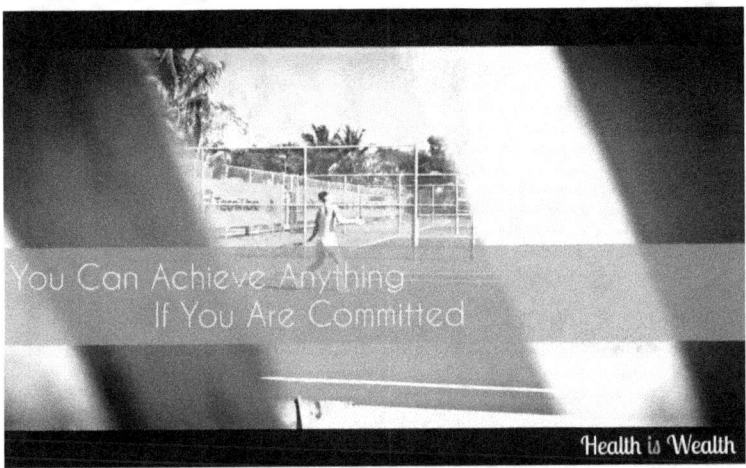

Are you interested or are you committed to achieving your current goals? Most may ask, what is the difference? If you have interest in fulfilling your goals, then you will complete your task and never look back. In other words, you will do things the same way as how most people do it. However, if you are committed to your situation, then you will find yourself working more than you need to, and trying to improve your current goals, although they are already good enough. Successful entrepreneurs are successful because they have a purpose behind their tasks, it is more than just interest. So just ask yourself, are you interested or are you committed to what you are currently doing.

There Should Never Be a Plan "B"

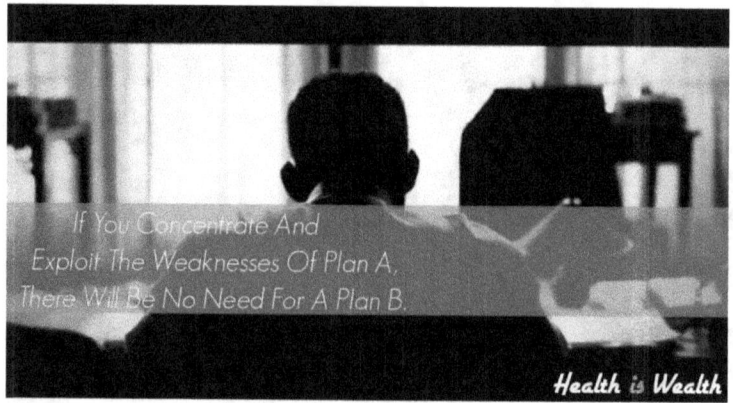

You've all heard of Plan B's. They are there to back you up just in case Plan A doesn't work. But what's the point of spending half your time on Plan A and half your time on Plan B. Instead, use your time to focus solely on Plan A so that you can perfect it. A perfect plan is better than two average plans. I've always grown up being told "If you do it right the first time, you won't have to do it a second time". So why do it a second time, you're just wasting energy. Perfect your 1st attempt so that you can move on and accomplish other things in life.

Become a Warrior

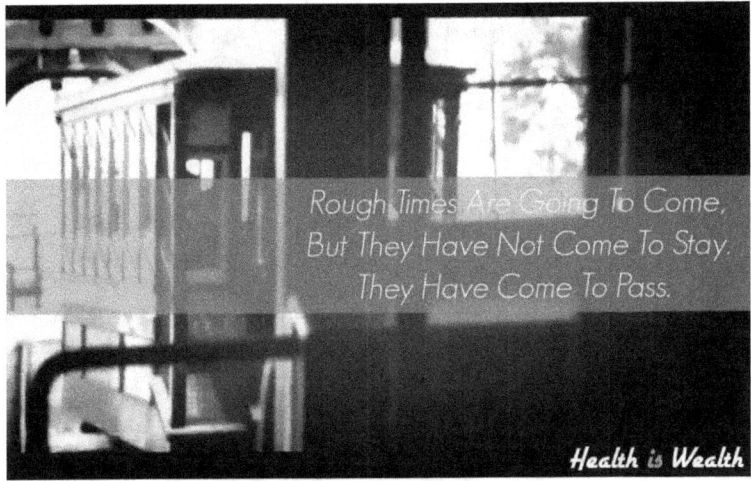

Rough Times Are Going To Come,
But They Have Not Come To Stay.
They Have Come To Pass.

Health is Wealth

It's not like we're never going to get hurt in life. And it's not like these episodes are meant to devastate us. These harsh times are just the flow of life and everyone gets them, we just need to do our part and accept them. It may sound easy but it really isn't. To accept tragedy or a mishap in your life is going to be hard because we're humans. We're emotional and that's understandable, but what about life. Life isn't going to wait for you, it's like a train with no brakes. The Sun is still going to shine, and the Moon is still going to glow. So try not to mourn for too long. These hard times are bound to come, but they have not come to stay. They have come to pass.

A Forgotten Lifestyle

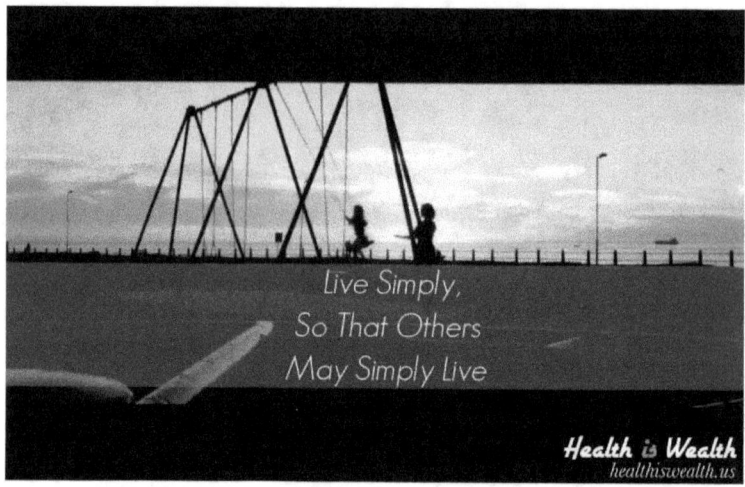

*Live Simply,
So That Others
May Simply Live*

Health is Wealth
healthiswealth.us

This is probably going to be my favorite for a while. Live simply, so that others may simply live. A simple saying that would do wonders for the world. In a world where capitalism is King, we often get carried away by lavish lifestyles that we envy of others. There's nothing wrong with treating yourself after a hard day's work. It's just that sometimes we become a bit too selfish. There are many people around us that aren't even able to even eat 3 times a day, and here we are complaining about getting the newest gadgets. Our job to live simply is not going to kill us. We may miss out on getting a few designer handbags or suits, but at the end of the day those funds will allow the unfortunate to live another day.

Stop Waiting and Just Do It

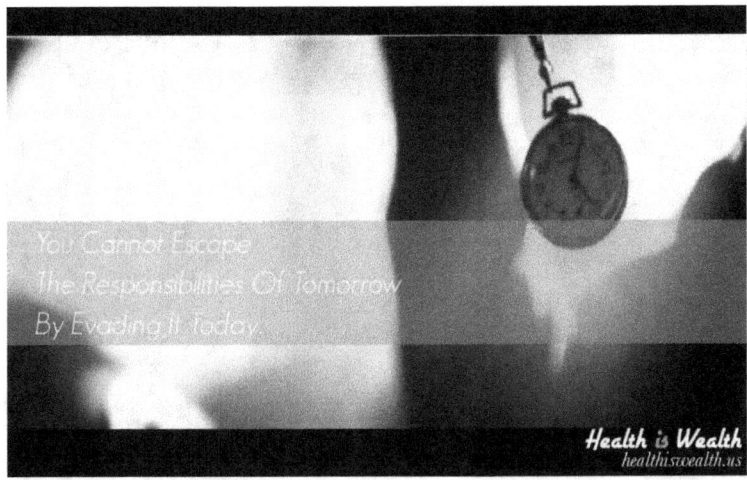

I'll do it later. For some reason we only feel obliged to start working when the deadline is near. Maybe you just need pressure to start working. We all put off work until later and our work becomes faulty when we're done. No time left to correct your mistakes. But that's not how successful people succeed and we need to instill in our minds to organize your workload so that you don't do last minute work.

You Are Only One Person, But...

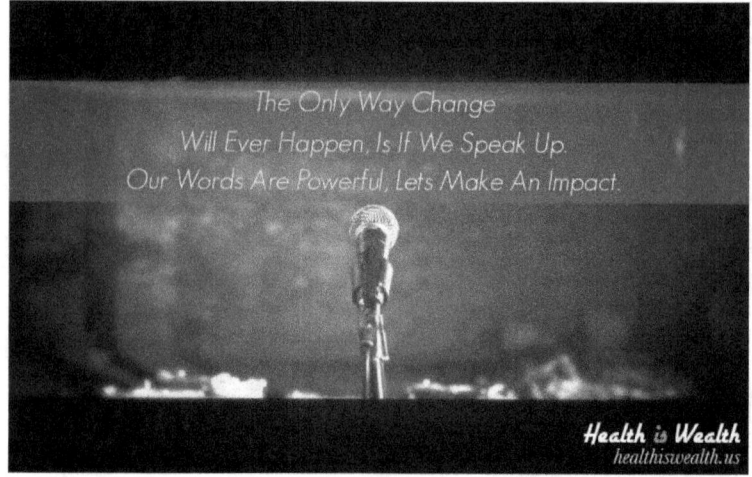

The Only Way Change
Will Ever Happen, Is If We Speak Up.
Our Words Are Powerful, Lets Make An Impact.

Health is Wealth
healthiswealth.us

This was always my problem. I'm guilty of the, "but I'm just one person" crime. I'm so used to assuming that other people are going to make an effort to change their surroundings that I suppose my input wouldn't make a difference. So what if you're just one person. If you're making a change and people around you see it, then they'll be inspired to make the change with you. You are never just one. There may be many others in the room who have the same idea as you, but are not confident enough to share. Stand up and speak your mind so that confidence may grow in them too. The only way change will ever happen, is if we speak up. Our words are powerful, let's make an impact. Don't ever think of yourself as just one.

My Dream Never Faded. Your Doubts Just made it More Clear to Me

They Asked Him, How Did He Do It?
He Replied,
There Was No One Here
To Tell Me I Couldn't Do It.

Health is Wealth

Are you sure? No one has ever done it before, so how will you do it? It's Impossible.

Well that's not new. People telling you what's possible and what's impossible. But what do they know. They don't know how much time and effort you put in every day and night into your work. If they tell you that it's impossible, let it fuel your fire. Proving people wrong was always a hobby of mine. So go out there and work. And when that day comes, you could tell your doubters that it was always possible.

Even if no one sees it for you, you must see it for yourself. And just like that you are on the road to success.

How's Your Willpower?

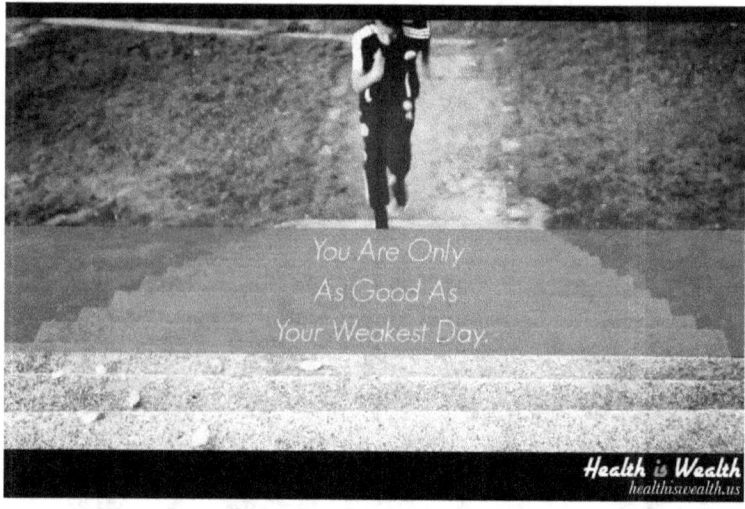

You Are Only
As Good As
Your Weakest Day.

Health is Wealth
healthiswealth.us

Stop setting goals and stopping half way. Sometimes we get inspired and decide to dream big. And after the next day the inspiration is gone and we decide to quit. The problem is not that we have set your goals too high. There's no such thing as setting your goals too high. The problem is us. If we don't want it bad enough, then we will be like the majority of people who start something and then say it's getting nowhere. Well don't expect results to come in just a couple of days, this is a long term commitment. We have to be committed to what we do in order to get far. We can start and end half way, but what does that really say about our willpower. You are only as good as your weakest day.

We Used to Dream a Lot

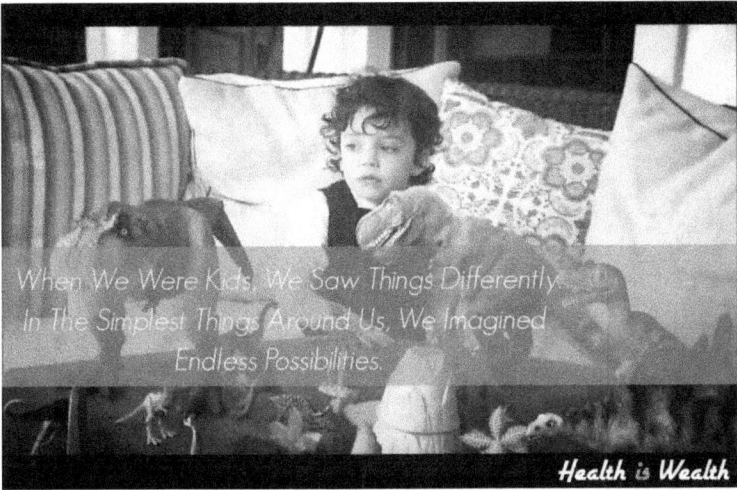

When We Were Kids, We Saw Things Differently.
In The Simplest Things Around Us, We Imagined
Endless Possibilities.

Health is Wealth

Back then we used to tie a towel around our neck and jump off our beds only to soar for a couple of seconds. But those couple of seconds were enough to allow us to feel like superheroes. We turned that towel into a cape and it gave us an identity. When we were kids, we saw things differently. In the simplest things around us, we imagined endless possibilities. Who would have known that a chunk of metal would help us fly around the world? That's absurd right? It's hard to imagine an airplane from looking at a chunk of metal. As we grow older we slowly push our imaginations aside, and that towel that used to help us fly is just a rag to us now. We've grown up in a world filled with pessimists, whom only know how to provide doubts into our imaginations. It's hard to be innovative when we have so much doubts in our own ideas. So just let those imaginations come back and give them another chance. You'll never know where those imaginations will take you.

G.R.I.N.D.

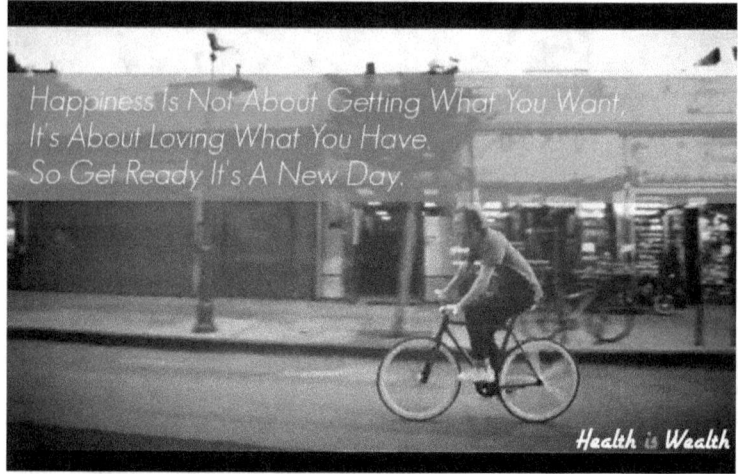

Sometimes I feel like I'm not making any progress toward my goals and it frightens me. My dreams and goals are still there, but I have my doubts like any human would. So today I turned on my speakers and Asher Roth was on. It was only then that I realized that I was doing it all wrong. My goal was to work hard so that I could buy my parents stuff that they would be happy to have. I wanted them to be happy. I wanted them to know that in the near future, their working hours would be lessened and that I would bombard them with gifts.

But it wasn't until today, that I realize how faulty my goals were. I was so focused on spending time on work for a better future that I nearly forgot about spending time with my parents in the present. Spending money on my parents can come a little later, but for now it's about spending time with the people you love. Happiness isn't not about getting what you want all the time, it's about loving what you have. So get ready, it's a new day.

Appreciate What You Have!

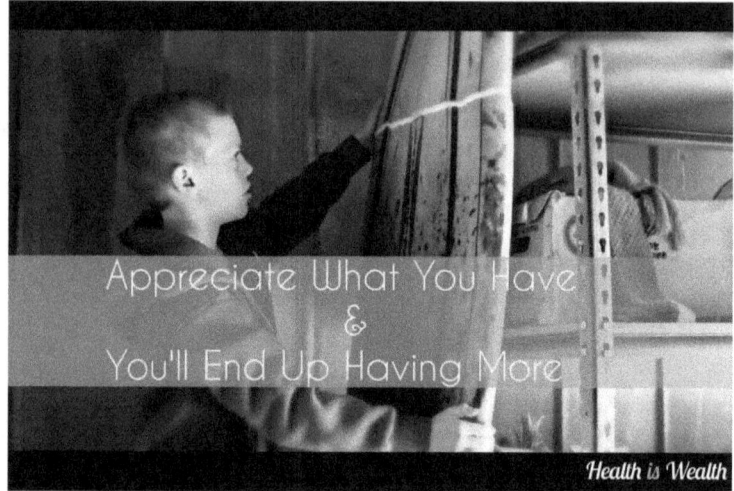

Appreciate What You Have
&
You'll End Up Having More

Health is Wealth

Today we are so focused with getting new things that we neglect what we already have. We look forward to creating new relationships, and leave behind the relationships we already have. Instead of trying to fix the problems in our current situations, we look for something new as a solution, but at the end of the day we are just dragging out the problem. So let's fix something today, before looking elsewhere. When a friendship is confronted with problems, they settle the problem with each other and grow stronger together.

Stuck in Your Comfort Zone?

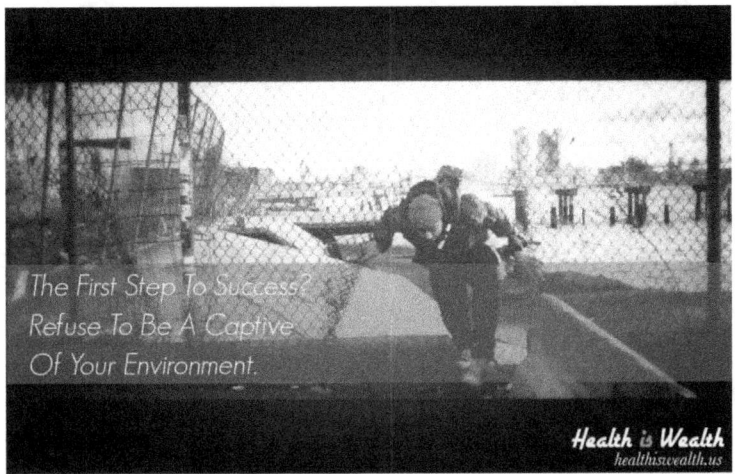

The First Step To Success?
Refuse To Be A Captive
Of Your Environment.

Health is Wealth
healthiswealth.us

You say you want to be healthy. You say you want to be rich. But are you doing anything towards these goals. Surrounding yourself with a room full of junk food is not going to help. Neither is hanging around people who don't believe in working hard. You need to get out of your old environment and go find a new one. Stop being trapped in the misery that is around you. Go meet new friends that actually care about the wellness of their body and people who set new goals every week. Once you are in their environment, you'll find yourself trying to work as hard as or even harder than them. Place yourself in a healthy environment, but first you have to leave your old one.

Thank you for taking the time to read this book and may you always have a perfectly balanced life. If you haven't already read my author's description before purchasing this book, you would know that I am also the founder of Finicky. The images provided by the book come from my website, "Finicky.us"

Preview of "Public Speaking: 7 Essentials Steps Used by Top Entrepreneurs"
You may purchase this book by clicking here

Or by using this link http://amzn.to/1dsxVg9

The feeling of nervousness or stage-fright when presenting to an audience is perfectly normal. Even the best public speakers still get nervous. This is a part of being human, we are wired to be worried about our reputation and public speaking is a threat to us. In psychological terms, our fight or flight responses comes into play and our body starts feeling different.

Before I go on any further, I would just like to tell you that the fears of public speaking are not to be overcome, we need to adapt to our public speaking environment. I would like you to keep this in mind as you continue to read on.

Before considering talking in public there are some things you must be aware of. The first thing you should do before speaking in public is to find out who you are and what you need.

The feedback you will receive after speaking in public is relevant for what you are going to do next. You should always meditate and answer these questions: Who am I? What do I want? What do I need?

www.ingramcontent.com/pod-product-compliance
Lightning Source LLC
Chambersburg PA
CBHW070829290526
45795CB00002B/884